Competency Based Fieldwork Evaluation

for Occupational Therapists

MANUAL

Ann Bossers, *M.Ed., OT (C), OT Reg. (Ont.)*
Linda T. Miller, *Ph.D.*
Helene J. Polatajko, *Ph.D., OT (C), OT Reg. (Ont.)*
Mark Hartley, *Hon BA Psych*

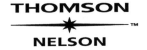

THOMSON

NELSON

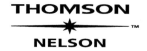

Printed and bound in Canada
8 9 10 11   12 11 10 09

For more information contact
Thomson Nelson
1120 Birchmount Road,
Scarborough, Ontario, M1K 5G4.
Or you can visit our internet site at
http://www.nelson.com

For permission to use material from this text or product, contact us by
Tel: 1-800-730-2214
Fax: 1-800-730-2215
www.thomsonrights.com

This textbook is a Nelson custom publication. Because your instructor has chosen to produce a custom publication, you pay only for material that you will use in your course.

ISBN-13 : 978-0-17-646538-4
ISBN-10 : 0-17-646538-3

Consists of Selections from:

Competency Based Fieldwork Evaluation for Occupational Therapists
Ann Bossers, Linda T. Miller, Helene J. Polatajko, Mark Hartley
ISBN-10: 0766873366

CONTENTS

PREFACE

Fieldwork is an integral part of all occupational therapy programs. Through the experiences provided in various settings and practice areas, students develop as occupational therapists. The Competency Based Fieldwork Evaluation for Occupational Therapists (CBFE-OT) is a measure designed to evaluate any level of fieldwork within all placement areas. The CBFE-OT is intended to be used by occupational therapy educational programs as the tool for both therapists and students to evaluate fieldwork.

The CBFE-OT captures current thinking in evaluation and is based on seven core competencies rather than the traditional long list of skills. These competencies include practice knowledge, clinical reasoning, facilitating change with a practice process, professional interactions and responsibility, communication, professional development, and performance management. The measure is easy to understand, user-friendly, and applicable in any setting, including both role-emerging and role-established placements. Incorporating adult learning principles, the CBFE-OT has an integrated learning contract for each of the seven competencies, which provides a way for the student to integrate his or her personalized learning objectives for each competency.

Development

The evaluation was developed by the authors through a lengthy period of study driven by the need to replace the skill-driven fieldwork evaluations that often lack relevancy for the diverse and evolving occupational therapy practice areas. The competency structure of the CBFE-OT allows for the flexibility to evaluate student performance across a wide range of settings and diverse occupational therapy roles, while reflecting the changing nature of health care practice. The evaluation scale is based on a developmental continuum and therefore can be used with a student at any fieldwork level. The CBFE-OT can be used with occupational therapy students from any university and is not tied to a particular curriculum model or program. Opportunities for self-directed learning are reinforced through the learning contract, which actively engages the student in developing personalized learning objectives, and by providing opportunities for learning within the fieldwork setting and the framework of the competencies.

Organization and Features

The CBFE-OT is comprised of a manual and an evaluation that is completed by the fieldwork educator and student. This book includes two copies of the evaluation for use in evaluating placements. Purchase of this book includes permission for the student to make additional copies of the evaluation for his/her additional placements.

The Manual

The manual is intended as a reference for the student, fieldwork educator, and degree-granting university. It provides an outline of the development of the instrument; instructions on how to evaluate competency development; a description of the developmental continuum, learning objectives, and the use of the contract; instructions for general use; criteria to determine pass/fail; and a glossary. The same manual can be used for all placements, and the student or university can ensure delivery of the manual to the placement site.

The Evaluation

The evaluation begins with a history sheet to record information describing the placement and space for the signatures of the student, fieldwork educator, and site practice leader. Following this sheet are pages for each of the seven competencies of practice. The educator in partnership with the student completes the evaluation at the placement midterm and final by indicating performance on each of the seven competency rating scales. Sections for narrative feedback at both the midterm and final are provided for each competency. In addition, a learning contract section is available for each competency. Below each contract is a visual analogue scale allowing the opportunity to rate progress on the objectives for the competency. The final page of the evaluation includes an overall rating scale, a section to identify future learning needs, and a box to indicate a recommendation of pass or fail. For each fieldwork placement a separate evaluation is used, and either the university or student ensures delivery of the evaluation form to the site.

Features

The CBFE-OT allows for evaluation of the student's performance by the student as well as the fieldwork evaluator, and can be kept on file at the university to help both the student and university track fieldwork competency over time and across practice areas. This tool is concise, focusing on core competencies, and is applicable to any level of fieldwork in any setting. In addition, student occupational therapists are encouraged to take ownership of their own professional development by creating personalized learning objectives, which can be used to guide their fieldwork experience.

ABOUT THE AUTHORS

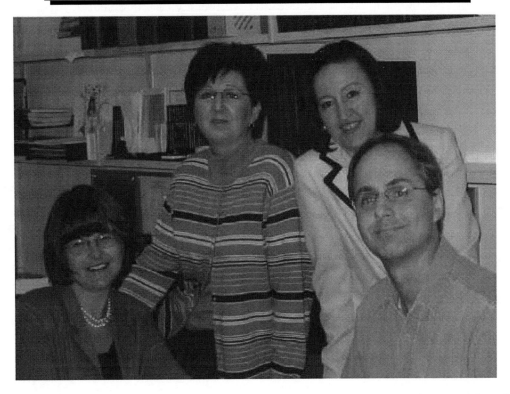

Ann Bossers, M.Ed., OT(C), OT Reg. (Ont.), is an Associate Professor and the Fieldwork Coordinator in the School of Occupational Therapy at The University of Western Ontario. She has held this position since 1987. Her publications, presentations, and workshops have focused on professionalism, mentorship, professional portfolios, and fieldwork. In addition to her peer-reviewed publications, she has written educational manuals on role-emerging fieldwork, interdisciplinary placements, student perceptions of the part-time therapist/full-time student fieldwork placement, and the student as supervisor model of fieldwork. Her ongoing research program continues to center on models of fieldwork, fieldwork evaluation, and fostering professionalism through a mentorship process. She has consulted with university programs, both nationally and internationally, regarding curriculum design and fieldwork integration.

Linda Miller received her Ph.D. in Psychology with a discipline specialty in Measurement from the Department of Psychology at The University of Western Ontario in 1994. Currently, she is a tenured Associate Professor in the School of Occupational Therapy at UWO. Dr. Miller's program of research is centered on measurement development and evaluation. Consistent with these interests, Dr. Miller's research has evolved to embrace the measurement of many rehabilitation phenomena, including cognitive abilities, language, motor performance, and clinical competencies. She has published 15 articles in a wide range of rehabilitation-related peer-reviewed journals since completing her Ph.D. Her work has been presented provincially, nationally, and internationally.

Helene Polatajko, Ph.D., OT(C), OT Reg. (Ont.), is Professor and Chair of the Department of Occupational Therapy at the University of Toronto. She also holds appointments with the Graduate Department of Rehabilitation Science, the Department of Public Health Science, and the School of Graduate Studies all at the University of Toronto, the Faculty of Graduate Studies at The University of Western Ontario, and the Department of Occupational Therapy, School of Health and Rehabilitation Sciences, the University of Queensland, Australia. She is an internationally acclaimed scholar in the fields of occupational therapy and developmental coordination disorder. She is an elected member of the American Academy of Research. Her major research has been in the areas of instrument development and treatment studies, and her major interest is in understanding and enabling occupation, particularly in children.

Mark Hartley, HonBA Psych., is a Research Associate in the School of Occupational Therapy at The University of Western Ontario. He has been an active member of the CBFE team since its inception in 1997. Currently, he is a member of a research team working on a project that is part of an international program of research examining theory and methods for assessing the psychosocial and quality-of-life impact of assistive devices for persons who have a physical disability. He has a solid academic background and extensive experience in research design, methods, and statistics, and has contributed a number of publications to the occupational therapy and neuroscience research literature.

ACKNOWLEDGMENTS

The authors wish to acknowledge the efforts of Arlene Anthony and Barbara Gaiptman who were members of the original team that developed the pilot version of the CBFE. In addition, we would like to thank the former London Life Insurance Company for providing us with a strong example of a competency based evaluation tool. A special word of thanks to Sandy Sargeant for her design contributions and to Jackie Klee for incorporating final changes in the manuscript. And a special note of thanks to the many therapists who contributed to the development and testing of the CBFE. From the initial focus groups, face validity checks, and pilot testing, therapists' feedback and ideas led to the development of the current tool. In addition, student input from living the experience and feedback provided to the research team have been very beneficial.

We extend grateful appreciation to McGill University and Laurie Snider, Caroline Storr, and Aliki Thomas in their support of the French translation of the CBFE and in collecting data on the CBFE.

Special thanks as well to Debra Cameron and Jill Stier and the University of Toronto for their role in collecting data on the use of the CBFE.

A special acknowledgment and thank you to the Ontario Council of University Programs (OCUPRS) for supporting the idea and the importance of a new fieldwork evaluation instrument and providing partial support to this project through grant dollars for clinical education provided to OCUPRS from the Ministry of Health. The university fieldwork coordinators from the University of Ottawa (School of Rehabilitation Sciences-Occupational Therapy and School of Communication Sciences and Disorders), the University of Toronto (Department of Occupational Therapy), and The University of Western Ontario (School of Physical Therapy and School of Occupational Therapy), through their role in disseminating the test materials in the pilot phase and helping the research group track the data in the initial stages of the project, have been greatly appreciated.

PREAMBLE

The modern tendency to evaluate health care as an economic concept has led to the restructuring of the health care system and to alterations in professional health care practice. Student evaluations designed prior to this recent social transition have rapidly become obsolete. In January 1997, researchers from The University of Western Ontario and the University of Toronto, with a grant from the Ontario Council of University Programs in Rehabilitation Sciences, undertook to develop a student evaluation that would incorporate the requisite set of abilities for therapists from the disciplines of audiology, physical therapy, occupational therapy, and speech language pathology. *The Competency Based Fieldwork Evaluation (CBFE) for Professional Rehabilitation Students* (Bossers, Miller, Polatajko, Hartley, Anthony, & Gaiptman, 1998) represented the culmination of their efforts. Further data collection resulted in the CBFE-OT.

Instrument Development

Development of the instrument was initiated in response to the changing nature of professional practice, and took into consideration new directions in community care and the consequent increase in development of community fieldwork sites (Bossers, Cook, Polatajko, & Laine, 1997; Gage, 1995; Pew Health Professions Commission, 1991). The first step in the development process was to determine the feasibility of creating an evaluation with applicability for all rehabilitation science students. Examination of a cross-section of evaluations from educational programs in North America, Europe, and Australia revealed that entry-level competence was described across the disciplines by a common set of competencies. One communicative disorders and one physical therapy assessment form were subsequently sent out to clinicians from another discipline. Therapists were asked to apply one of the forms to a same discipline student and rate the relative validity of each descriptor (e.g., a CD student was evaluated by a CD clinician using a PT evaluation). Feedback from clinicians tended to confirm that the requisite abilities for entry-level therapists in all disciplines were described by a core set of common competencies.

After establishing the validity of evaluating students across disciplines with a standard evaluation, the research group began the task of formally delineating the domain of competence for rehabilitation therapists. A representative list of the competencies were assessed by a large cross-section of evaluations from all disciplines was compiled and then edited through a process of discussion; redundant or inappropriate items were removed, and new competencies were added. The revised list was cross-referenced with recently published standards of practice and determined to be a comprehensive representation of the domains of competence. Input received from therapists in a wide range of practice areas, gathered through two different focus groups, along with data collected from participants of the CD/PT pilot, were incorporated into the form's design.

The form's contents were given an organizational structure. After examining the assessment systems used by various programs, the domain of competence for rehabilitation therapists was inserted into a format similar to that of the London Life Core Competency Evaluation form (London Life Insurance Company, 1994). This London Life document was created to guide employees in the development of occupational competence, and as a system for evaluating employee performance. The design facilitated comprehensive, timely, and accurate evaluation in diverse settings. The research group experimented with several prototype rating scales before designing a customized Competency Rating Scale. The form's components were assembled into a cohesive document, copies of the CBFE were distributed to experienced members of the clinical community for review, and the evaluation was revised on the basis of results from the face validity pilot.

A second pilot study evaluated the CBFE's ability to measure student performance and competency development. The design was cross-sectional and comparative, involving the occupational therapy, physical therapy, and communicative disorder disciplines. Therapists evaluated students using the CBFE as well as their existing evaluation tool. Both therapists and students completed a questionnaire regarding the usage of the CBFE. Findings from this study (Miller, Bossers, Polatajko, & Hartley, 2001) were used to amend the document and have resulted in the final version of the CBFE-OT.

Results of the Miller et al. (2001) pilot study indicated that the CBFE accurately reflected the development of students across placement levels. Further, correlations between the CBFE competencies and a currently widely used fieldwork evaluation instrument for occupational therapy students indicated some overlap in the constructs measured by the two instruments. However, the lack of consistently high correlations between the two instruments suggests that the CBFE is measuring information beyond what is obtained in the other instrument. This distinct information is likely related to the CBFE's focus on global competencies, rather than specific skills, and its relevance across a wide range of placement settings.

The CBFE and, in particular, the competencies included in the CBFE-OT, have been recognized by the Association of Canadian Occupational Therapy Regulatory Organizations (ACOTRO) as a framework to capture the competencies required for practice as an occupational therapist (OT) in Canada (ACOTRO, 2000). The ACOTRO competencies for occupational therapists closely parallel those identified in the CBFE. Both identify seven competencies that are essentially the same but are named slightly differently. The outcome of the national validation process conducted by ACOTRO offers strong evidence of the validity of the CBFE competency model; the CBFE is based on a model of competencies consistent with the expectations for competence in practicing occupational therapists.

INTRODUCTION

Performance is the observable outcome of a set of specific causes and influences. In the business field, Prahadad and Hamel (1990) introduced the concept of "core competencies" related to the global organization versus attributes at the individual level. Over the past decade definitions of competency in the literature vary (Shippman, 2000). Within the CBFE, competence is regarded as the capacity to conceptualize and operationalize the performance necessary for a certain type of outcome in a given situation. Competency defines, in behavioral terms, the adequate performance of different activities. Professional competency is the behavioral definition of the knowledge, skills, behaviors, values, and personal characteristics that underlie the adequate performance of professional activities. Professional competence is a capacity that human societies create and impart to groups of individuals who are then entrusted to utilize their gifts for the public good and to sustain the growth of their profession. An essential responsibility of those in the health care profession is to ensure clients receive safe and effective service. Student evaluation is central to meeting this responsibility; assessment of a student's fieldwork performance efficaciously guides the development of professional competence and ensures the student is qualified for professional practice.

Ensuring a Student Is Qualified to Enter Professional Practice

Students develop the requisite set of competencies characteristic of an entry-level therapist by completing a specially designed program of formal education. To graduate from an accredited program, a student must attain a level of professional competence equal to that of an entry-level clinician. Determining if a student meets this criterion is an objective procedure. The performance required of an entry-level clinician is defined in terms of clear, objective, measurable outcomes by experienced members of the profession, and a student's fieldwork performance is measured in terms of how closely it compares to the behavioral definition of entry-level competence. The measurement is all that is needed to determine whether the student is competent to enter practice. For example, if the behavioral definition of numerical competence is "scoring 90% on a standardized, written test of arithmetic," then a test score is a measure of a student's performance or level of competency, and only students who score 90% or higher are numerically competent. A fieldwork educator's assessment of the short-term behavior exhibited by a student on placement is sufficient for determining entry-level competence because each student's performance is compared to the same standard (i.e., the

1

behavioral definition of entry-level competence). Although competence is an abstraction that cannot be measured directly, a student's behavior (or performance) can be interpreted as a valid index of his or her level of competency.

Evaluating a Student's Professional Competency Development

Student evaluation has a second important purpose that is more difficult to achieve. Throughout the educational program, both educator and learner must monitor the student's progress to ensure that development proceeds within parameters established by the profession. A formal assessment of a student's level of competence relative to an entry-level clinician's competence provides a profile of development that can serve as a basis for evaluating the student's current level of progress and for prudently directing future learning. Determining competence to enter practice is the first step in evaluating developmental progress. The former is an objective measurement (of a student's level of competency) based on a comparison between two performances (the student's clinical performance and the behavioral definition of the performance of an entry-level clinician) and the latter is a standardized interpretation of the measurement. To assess a student's level of progress, the measurement of clinical performance is evaluated within the context of the student's previous learning opportunities, the nature of the competence being evaluated, and the normal pattern of long-run development. This process involves the student, the fieldwork educator/supervisor, and the university program.

Why Evaluating Progress Requires Interpreting the Measure of Student Performance

The developmental process is an ongoing interaction between a person's unique characteristics and the educational experiences provided by the curriculum of a particular school. In addition, what can be learned in any current situation is dependent upon past learning. This means that the course of development on a day-to-day, week-to-week, or month-to-month basis will vary across individuals, as will the observable expression of learning. Therefore, evaluating developmental progress requires comparing a supervisor's assessment of a student's performance to a subjective, but systematically defined, individual standard.

The subjective standard of comparison for each individual student takes into consideration past learning, the current learning situation, and the global pattern of development. In the long run, the course of development follows a global pattern. Students exposed to a particular set of conditions (the curriculum) tend to reach a certain level of development (entry-level clinician) within a specific time range (the length of the program). The behavior of students who advance through the curriculum varies predictably as they gain knowledge and experience. This means that students typically perform in characteristic ways at different stages of development (Chambers & Glassman, 1997).

The developmental stages proposed have not been empirically validated but are based on theoretical reasoning and are believed to provide a strong framework for assessing student development. Figure 1 provides an illustration of the developmental stages of professional development.

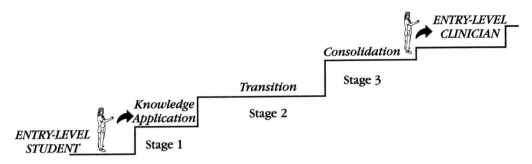

Figure 1 Stages of Professional Competency Development

Entry-Level Student

Entry-level or beginning students are introduced to basic concepts of professional practice in the classroom and to the clinical environment during fieldwork placements. Initially, they may approach these areas as separate domains of learning. Students on their first placement are often occupied with becoming familiar with the dynamics of a fieldwork setting. They have not had time to develop the knowledge and problem-solving skills necessary for independent action within the fieldwork environment. Consider the analogy of novice drivers. Learning the rules of the road and learning to physically drive a car are separate activities; a person can become competent in one of these areas without becoming competent in the other. Developing the competence of a licensed driver is the process of learning to apply the rules of the road while driving the car.

Early on, students' fieldwork may focus on the application of academic knowledge without simultaneous consideration of environmental feedback (Neistadt, 1996). Entry-level students may be uncomfortable with the idea that there could be more than one solution to a problem. Entry-level students who have been prepared for the complexities of the fieldwork environment during coursework are motivated to learn, have developed learning abilities and a clear conception of what is required of them, are able to identify the need for further information and ask appropriate questions, and can identify and reflect upon personal strengths and weaknesses.

With most students, at any stage of development, there is an initial period of adaptation as students enter new areas of practice.

Knowledge Application

Soon after entry level, students begin the task of acquiring the body of knowledge and repertoire of skills necessary for professional practice. As they move through the curriculum and gain experience in the clinical environment, students learn the principles of practice and become familiar with the role of their discipline. During this stage of development, students need to observe, practice skills, and reflect on their performance.

Providing direct evaluation and feedback is useful for beginning students with little or no fieldwork experience or for students who are inexperienced in a specific area of practice (Anderson, 1988). Students need an opportunity to take an active role working with clients to apply their knowledge, and to develop and practice interaction, assessment, intervention, and professional reasoning skills. They are becoming familiar with the roles of the therapist (Sullivan & Bossers, 1998).

Transition

Transition (Anderson, 1988) is a developmental stage between knowledge application and consolidation. Although students at this stage interact with their fieldwork educator to varying degrees to solve problems or make decisions, they are able to make meaningful contributions as members of a health care team.

The emphasis during this developmental stage is on practice and experience in problem solving, assessment, and intervention. Students begin to share and assume responsibility for all components of practice. Students should be encouraged to try to develop their own ideas and insights regarding clients, engage in discussion of solutions to clinical problems, and begin to make decisions about the most viable course of action. Students should be encouraged to engage in self-analysis and reflection and to share and integrate previous learning experiences into their practice (Sullivan & Bossers, 1998).

The Coaching Supervision Strategy (Hagler & McFarlane, 1991) is appropriate for students in the process of developing autonomy and independence. A coach is a highly supportive role model who intercedes in difficult situations to collaboratively solve problems while gradually increasing a student's responsibility for professional decision making (Gaiptman & Anthony, 1993).

Consolidation

Consolidation (Sullivan & Bossers, 1998) is the final stage of student development. It is expected that students near the end of the curriculum will have already internalized the core body of specialized knowledge, skills, and values that form the basis of professional practice. They should be able to accurately analyze and appropriately alter their own behavior, solve problems independently, and function effectively in the fieldwork environment without continuous observation or evaluation. However, students in the consolidation stage continue to interact with experienced clinicians to further their development as professionals.

The Consultation Supervision Strategy is appropriate for students who have reached the consolidation stage. Consultation is essentially a "helping process that emerges out of a need to solve a problem" (Anderson, 1988). The fieldwork educator assists a student with a specific problem by collaborating as a peer to generate potential solutions.

Entry-Level Clinician

An entry-level clinician is a graduate from an accredited program who is entering practice as a therapist.

The Competency Rating Scale

The stages of development are incorporated in a rating scale known as a Competency Rating Scale (CRS), as illustrated in Figure 2. A student's development is conceptualized as taking place along a continuum that spans the duration of the curriculum. Development begins when a student enters an educational program (point on the scale labeled "Entry-Level Student"), progresses along the scale through three stages (knowledge application, transition, and consolidation), and concludes at graduation when the student is deemed to be qualified to enter professional practice (point on the scale labeled "Entry-Level Clinician"). More globally, the developmental continuum of a professional continues throughout a therapist's professional career.

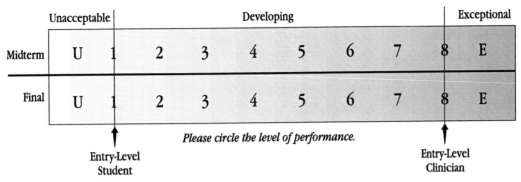

Figure 2   The Competency Rating Scale

The CRS allows fieldwork educators to rate a student's level of professional competence. The two endpoints of the scale (Entry-Level Student and Entry-Level Clinician) are upper and lower limits that delineate the qualitative range of behavior measured by the scale. Performances qualitatively outside these boundaries indicate variation from the description of developmental progression. Unusually inadequate performances are "red flags" for taking remedial action with a student. Exceptionally competent performances index high-ability students. (Refer to Table 1 for the definitions of the stages of competency development.) Fieldwork educators should circle the number on the scale that best represents their judgment of a student's characteristics in relation to either scale endpoint.

Learning Objectives

The evaluation form identifies seven competencies. Throughout the placement, students will be working on developing their knowledge, attitudes, and skills in all domains, and will be evaluated on all seven competencies. However, as students reflect on their previous experiences and learning needs, they identify areas in which they wish to focus their learning during placement. Students develop learning objectives that blend these identified learning needs with the requirements of the professional education program and the learning opportunities available at the placement.

By developing their own learning objectives, the students can individualize their learning program and make explicit the areas on which they will focus. It is not necessary that students develop objectives for each of the seven competencies in the evaluation form.

Table 1: Definitions of Stages of Student Professional Competency Development

	Developing		
Student Performance	Knowledge Application	Transition-Reflection on Action	Consolidation-Reflection in Action
Supervision Style	Direct Teaching/ Evaluation/Feedback	Coaching	Consulting/ Mentoring

Table 2: Description of Components of a Learning Contract

1. Learning Objective(s)	2. Learning Resource	3. Evidence	4. Validation
What do you want to learn or develop? Consider your own competency levels and the opportunities available within this agency.	What will you utilize to achieve your learning objective(s)? Where can you find information? Be specific; consider how you learn best.	How can you demonstrate that you have met your learning objective(s)? What proof will you offer and when?	How do you want your evidence to be evaluated? By whom? When? What are the criteria for evaluation?

The Learning Objective Rating Scale

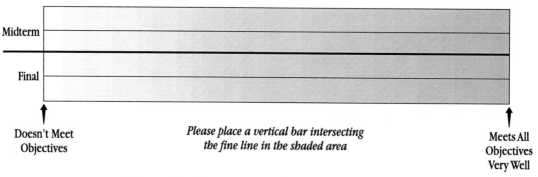

Figure 3   The Learning Objective Rating Scale

Developing the learning objectives is a dynamic process that involves discussion, negotiation, and collaboration among students and between students and fieldwork educators. For each objective that is developed, students will indicate what they want to learn or develop ("Objective[s]"), the learning resources and strategies that they will utilize to meet their learning objective(s) ("Resources"), the evidence that will demonstrate that they have met the objective(s) ("Evidence"), and the criteria by which the evidence will be evaluated ("Validation"). (See Table 2 for a description of the components of a learning contract and Figure 3 for the Learning Objective Rating Scale.)

Instructions for Completing Student Evaluation

1. This competency based evaluation form is designed for use in evaluating fieldwork/clinical placements for occupational therapy students. The student and fieldwork educator will establish learning objectives and evaluate the performance expected of a student occupational therapist within the particular practice area.

2. The competencies and their domains are described in Table 3.

3. The student formulates personal learning objectives that reflect his or her individual learning needs.

4. The therapist is to rate each competency using the Competency Rating Scale. Should the therapist wish to rate the student's performance on the learning objective, a second scale, the

Table 3: The Competencies of the CBFE-OT

Competency	Domain of Competency
1. Practice Knowledge	Discipline-specific theory and technical knowledge.
2. Clinical Reasoning	Analytical and conceptual thinking, judgment, decision making, and problem solving.
3. Facilitating Change with a Practice Process	Assessment, intervention planning, intervention delivery, and discharge planning.
4. Professional Interactions and Responsibility	Relationship with clients and colleagues, legal and ethical standards.
5. Communication	Verbal, nonverbal, and written communication.
6. Professional Development	Commitment to profession, self-directed learning, and accountability.
7. Performance Management	Time and resource management, leadership.

Learning Objectives Rating Scale (Figure 3) is provided. This is a visual analogue scale and the therapist can place a line anywhere along the scale.

5. The rating scale, as illustrated in Figure 2, covers a range from "unacceptable" to "exceptional."

6. Ratings are made for midterm evaluation by circling the number in the upper portion of the rating box (above the horizontal line). For final evaluation, circle the number in the lower portion of the rating box (below the horizontal line). It is expected that most students will perform in the "developing" range, between "Entry-Level Student" and "Entry-Level Clinician." A rating of "Unacceptable" should be used when a student's knowledge is lacking or actions are inappropriate, improper, incorrect, or unsafe. A rating of "Entry-Level Clinician" is used when a student demonstrates the performance of a newly hired recent graduate (an individual may not have experience in a broad range of settings or with complex cases). A rating of "exceptional" should be used when a student demonstrates the knowledge and performance of an experienced therapist. (Refer to Table 4 for the definitions of the stages of competency development.)

The "developing" range spans from the student's introduction to the field to the period of transition and ultimately consolidation. Progression along the "developing" range is exemplified by increased speed and efficiency in practice, increased knowledge, better reasoning, and decreased observation time. Educator strategies move from direct evaluation feedback to coaching and the encouragement of reflection on action, to a consultative model of supervision and fostering reflection in action (Anderson, 1988; McFarlane & Hagler, 1995; Schön, 1987).

7. Therapists are to consider the descriptors when rating each competency and when formulating comments.

8. Throughout the evaluation, reference is made to the "client." "Client" refers to individual clients, client groups, or families of clients.

9. The glossary at the end of the tool further defines the terms used throughout the CBFE-OT.

10. To facilitate the development of self-evaluation skills, the CBFE-OT can be completed by the student, as well as by the supervising therapist. Student self-evaluation may also facilitate the identification of future learning objectives.

11. To determine passing grades, academic programs establish criteria consistent with their curriculum. The CBFE-OT competency ratings, qualitative comments, and the fieldwork educator's recommendation of pass/fail are all considered. (See the Appendix for a more detailed description of pass/fail criteria and data collected from several Canadian university programs.)

Table 4: Definition of the Stages of Competency Development

DEFINITIONS FOR STAGES OF STUDENT PROFESSIONAL COMPETENCY DEVELOPMENT		
DEVELOPING		
	STAGE 1	*STAGE 2*	*STAGE 3*
Student Performance	Knowledge Application	Transition—Reflection on Action	Consolidation—Reflection in Action
Educator Supervision Style	Direct Teaching/ Evaluation/Feedback	Coaching	Consulting/Mentoring
Scoring	**Scores 1–3** 1 = low Stage 1 competencies 2 = rudimentary Stage 1 competencies 3 = mastery of Stage 1 competencies/ transition to Stage 2	**Scores 3–6** 3 = transition to Stage 2 4 = rudimentary Stage 2 competencies 5 = intermediate Stage 2 competencies 6 = mastery of Stage 2 competencies/transition to Stage 3	**Scores 6–8** 6 = transition to Stage 3 7 = rudimentary Stage 8 = mastery of Stage 3 competencies/ready to enter clinical practice

Appendix:
Establishing Criteria for Pass/Fail on Fieldwork Placements

The Competency Based Fieldwork Evaluation for Occupational Therapists is intended for use in evaluating students' performance in fieldwork placements. Ultimately, it is necessary to determine whether a student's performance qualifies for a passing grade in the fieldwork placement, necessitating the designation of a cutoff, for a pass. Because professional programs vary in their curricula and the timing and duration of fieldwork placements within their curricula, it is not possible to designate national, or cross-curricula, criteria for a passing grade. Alternatively, it is recommended that programs develop their own criteria for a passing grade that are consistent with the development of students within their own curriculum. The process of establishing "local cutoffs" necessitates the collection of data from students within a program over the course of several years, in order to establish patterns of performance across the placement levels. During the initial period of using the instrument without the benefit of local norms, it is recommended that determination of a passing grade be made with consideration given to the qualitative comments included in the form, and to the fieldwork educator's recommendation of a pass or fail.

It is recommended that local, or program-specific, cutoffs be established by cumulating scores obtained on the CBFE-OT for each placement within a curriculum over a period of three years. The three-year data set can then be used to calculate descriptive statistics for each competency and the average across the seven competencies for each placement level. These descriptive statistics would then reflect the average performance and variability in performance for each placement level based on three years of student data within the curriculum. The mean performance on the competencies reflects the average, or expected, performance, and scores above and below the mean reflect superior and subaverage performance, respectively. The standard deviation can be used to identify performance that is unacceptably below average. Based on the properties of the normal distribution, 6.68% of all students would be expected to obtain a rating that is 1.5 standard deviation units, or more, below the group mean; only 2.28% would be expected to obtain a score that is 2 standard deviation units, or more, below the group mean. Therefore, criteria can be established based on the number of standard deviation units that a score can fall below the group mean.

Table 5 is a summary of pilot data collected from three occupational therapy programs in Canada. The CBFE-OT was used to evaluate students at various placement levels, as indicated by the number of fieldwork hours. The sample used to calculate the mean and standard deviation varies across the placement levels based on the particular placement level used for piloting of the instrument. The average of the seven competencies for each student evaluated was used in the calculation of the level means. These data are provided to illustrate the use of means and standard deviations derived from cumulated data for the determination of passing criteria. Consider, for example, the Level 1 Placement with 150 fieldwork hours; the group mean of the average of the seven competencies is 3.57, with a standard deviation of 1.06. By calculating 1.5 standard deviations below the mean,

$$3.57 - (1.5 \times 1.06) = 1.98$$

a passing score of 1.98 would be obtained. Use of this criterion would imply that a score of 1.98, or less, is unacceptable; this suggests that the performance of the lowest 6.68% of the norming group (i.e., the three-year cumulated group) is unacceptable. Alternatively, by calculating 2 standard deviations below the mean,

Table 5: Using Means and Standard Deviations in the Estimation of Passing Criteria

Placement Level	Cumulative Number of Fieldwork Hours at Placement Completion	*N*	Number of Programs Included	*Mean*	*SD*	−1.5 *SD*	−2 *SD*
1	150 hrs*	90	1	3.57	1.06	1.98	1.45
1	240 hrs*	98	2	3.49	1.11	1.83	1.27
2	480 hrs	129	2	6.09	0.8	4.89	4.49
3 (Initial)	720 hrs**	92	2	6.89	1.02	5.36	4.85
3 (Final)	1020 hrs**	37	1	7.98	0.53	7.19	6.92

*The 150 hour and 240 hour placements are both Level 1 placements, differing only in length.

**Both of these placements are classified as Level 3 placements; however, the 720 hour placement is considered to reflect the beginning of Level 3 development, whereas the 1020 hour placement reflects the final stages of Level 3.

$$3.57 - (2.0 \times 1.06) = 1.45$$

a passing score of 1.45 would be obtained. This criterion would imply that a score of 1.45, or less, is unacceptable, suggesting that the performance of the lowest 2.28% of the norming group is unacceptable.

Table 5 provides an illustration of the use of standard deviation units to derive passing criteria across the levels. Although these data are illustrative and could provide a reference for the interpretation of scores over the initial three-year period of cumulating data, they should not be used as the passing criteria for specific programs. Because the data below have been cumulated across three different programs, they may not reflect the variations inherent in the individual curricula.

It is interesting to note that, even when combining data across programs, a clear pattern of score progression is apparent. A single factor analysis of variance was applied to these data to test for significance across the placement levels. A significant placement level effect was found $[F(4,441) = 324.31, < 0.001]$ and post hoc comparisons, using Tukey's procedure, revealed significant differences in performance among all placements, with the exception of the two Level 1 placements (150 hours versus 240 hours), indicating the longer Level 1 placement did not lead to significantly higher CBFE-OT scores. These data indicate that the average of the seven CBFE-OT competencies increases significantly across the placement levels, reflecting significant improvements in students' performance with increasing placement level. To further evaluate the relationship between placement level and CBFE-OT scores, a correlation was calculated between the cumulative number of fieldwork hours and average score across the seven competencies for each placement. A Pearson correlation of 0.83 was obtained, indicating a strong relationship between the number of hours of fieldwork experience and average CBFE-OT performance.

GLOSSARY

Adapts to Change The person's behavioral responses to changes in the workplace are shaped by thoughtful consideration of the purposes, goals, and best interests of the organization as a whole.

Advocates Actively supports and promotes the legitimate cause of another without regard for the popularity of her or his actions

Analytical Thinking A thought process for forming an insightful, comprehensive, mental representation of a complex problem or situation. Requires defining the whole problem in terms of its parts (i.e., considering each component part as a separate problem and finding its cause) and then defining the parts in terms of the whole problem (i.e., identifying how all other parts contribute to the cause of each individual part) in order to understand the cause-and-effect relationships within and between the elements that combine to form the problem.

Client-Centered View that people are intrinsic, interrelated parts of the environmental systems they inhabit; each person's subjective experience of being in the environment is unique, and a person's overall state of health must be understood as a complex interaction among the physical, mental, social, and spiritual factors that comprise human existence.

Colleagues Professional associates and other personnel cooperating to provide health care to clients.

Competence The type or quality of performance necessary to function properly in a given situation, expressed in terms of clear, measurable, objective outcomes that implicitly or explicitly define the knowledge, skills, values, and personal characteristics required to produce the performance.

Competency An actual performance indicative of an individual's capacity to function competently in a given situation. A performance measured in terms of how closely it compares to competence.

Professional Competency The behavioral definition of the knowledge, skills, values, and personal qualities that underlie the adequate performance of professional activities.

Competency Based Evaluation Competency based evaluation is a method of assessing an individual's ability to perform or demonstrate identified behaviors according to established criteria while achieving desirable outcomes under the varied circumstances of the real world (Benner, 1982).

Conceptual Thinking Conceptual thinking is the process of linking objective features of a situation to past learning. *Example:* Because red lights are features of many situations, determining how to respond to a specific occurrence of a red light requires conceptual thinking. For example, most Canadians or Americans would interpret a red light, at the top of a yellow pole, situated on a traffic island in a busy intersection as a signal to stop. Someone from a remote tribal culture would probably interpret the situation quite differently. The meaning people attribute to the red light would be derived from the meanings they attributed to various other features of the situation. The meaning people assigned to each feature would depend on their knowledge of phenomena similar to the component features of the current situation and the way they applied this information. (The meaning attributed to each individual feature of the situation may also depend on the various meanings attributed to the other features of the situation.) Correct interpretation of the "red light" scenario leads to the correct response, to stop.

Clinical reasoning employs conceptual thinking. Conceptual thinking has a logical structure: individual features of clients' situations can be related to a body of professional knowledge. The clinical reasoning process involves organizing information gleaned through conceptual thinking into a logically related framework, forming the most appropriate clinical interpretation of the situation, and responding to the client's needs on the basis of the interpretation. Sound clinical reasoning often points out an appropriate response.

Coaching   A supervision strategy appropriate for students in the process of developing autonomy and independence. A coach is a highly supportive role model who intercedes in difficult situations to collaboratively solve problems while gradually increasing a student's responsibility for professional decision making as her or his skill level improves.

Consolidation   The final stage of student development. It is expected that students near the end of the curriculum will have internalized the core body of specialized knowledge, procedures, skills, and values that form the basis of professional practice. They should be able to

accurately analyze and appropriately alter their own behavior, solve problems independently, and function effectively in the fieldwork environment without continuous observation or evaluation. However, students in the consolidation stage can consult and collaborate with experienced clinicians to practice and develop as professionals.

Consultation   A supervision strategy appropriate for advanced students who have reached the consolidation stage. Consultation is essentially a "helping process that emerges out of a need to solve a problem" (Anderson, 1988). A supervisor assists a student with a specific problem by collaborating as a peer to generate potential solutions. The fieldwork educator's role consists mainly of listening, supporting, and problem solving, but may also include giving direct suggestions.

Core Values   The foundational values, purposes, belief systems, and guiding principles that shape practice.

Developing Range   A student's development is conceptualized as taking place along a continuum that spans the duration of the curriculum. Development begins when a student enters an educational program (point on the scale labeled "Entry-Level Student"), progresses along the continuum through three stages (knowledge application, transition, and consolidation), and concludes at graduation when the student is deemed to be qualified to enter professional practice (point on the scale labeled "Entry-Level Clinician"). More globally, the developmental continuum of a professional continues throughout a therapist's professional career.

Direct Evaluation Feedback Supervision Strategy   A supervision strategy appropriate for students in the early stages of development. The strategy is useful for beginning students with little or no fieldwork experience or for students who are inexperienced in a specific area of practice. Fieldwork educators working with students at the knowledge application stage often engage in direct teaching, evaluation, and feedback.

Entry-Level Clinician A graduate from an accredited program who is entering practice as a therapist.

Entry-Level Student Entry level is a brief period when a student first enters an educational program. An experienced student endeavoring to learn a new area of practice, however, can also be expected to demonstrate behaviors and characteristics similar to those of an inexperienced student. The more advanced a student is, however, the less his or her performance should be affected by inexperience. Students nearing the end of the curriculum should be able to demonstrate acceptable performance in most situations.

Exceptional When a student demonstrates the knowledge and performance of an experienced clinician.

Facilitating Change Facilitating change refers to "all acts focused on change, including initiating, responding to, managing, advocating for, adopting to, and shaping change. This includes, but is not limited to, more traditional concepts of therapeutic intervention. Change may occur in the person, the occupation, the environment, or in any combination of these" (Landry, Hobson, & Polatajko, 1997).

Knowledge Application Soon after entry level, students begin the task of acquiring the body of knowledge and repertoire of skills necessary for professional practice. As they move through the curriculum and gain experience in the clinical environment, students learn the principles of practice and become familiar with the role of their discipline. During this stage of development, students need to observe and practice skills.

Leadership A leader guides, directs, and acts as a catalyst for new learning and improved performance in others, or seeks to learn and improve his or her own performance by diligently following the direction and guidance of more accomplished peers.

Learning Objectives Well-defined, measurable activities designed to increase or improve a student's knowledge, attitudes, or skills.

Operational and Organizational Awareness A working knowledge of the functional (the purpose, location, and rules of procedure of the various departments and specialized personnel that cooperate to achieve the purposes of the organization) and administrative structure (the hierarchy of responsibility for decision making) of the agencies and professional bodies relevant to practice. Awareness of the policies, procedures, and processes that must be followed when engaging in hands-on practice in a facility or when undertaking a specific professional role.

Parameters of the Profession The responsibilities and limits of professional practice. In other words, where the role of the profession begins and ends within the health care system.

Professional Integrity Firm adherence to the conduct, values, and qualities that characterize the profession.

Quality Management The continuous process of ensuring that the quality of service provided to clients is in keeping with the highest standards of the health care profession.

Reflection in Action When individuals critically analyze what they are doing while they are doing it, and simultaneously use the results of this analysis to improve the efficacy of their action without interrupting its expression.

Reflection on Action A personal, retrospective analysis of a subjective experience for the purpose of finding ways to improve the efficacy of one's own behavior in similar, future situations. When students mentally represent and analyze the actions they took while performing clinical activities or during interpersonal interactions within the fieldwork environment, they deepen their understanding of professional behavior.

Rehabilitation Student A person enrolled in an accredited audiology, occupational therapy, physical therapy, or speech language pathology program for the purpose of becoming a qualified therapist.

Resource Utilization Safe, efficient, and effective use of human, financial, and material resources.

Supervision Strategy The style or mode of supervisor/student interaction appropriate for the skill level and learning style of an individual student.

Supervising Therapist A therapist who educates, supervises, and evaluates a same discipline student. This term can be considered synonymous with "fieldwork educator" or "preceptor."

Technical Expertise The ability to perform the skilled activities necessary for professional practice with proficiency, in response to the demands of any given situation.

Theoretical Knowledge A thorough understanding of the system of assumptions, accepted principles, and rules of procedure that serve as blueprints for a specific manner of organizing knowledge to guide practice.

Transition A developmental stage between knowledge application and consolidation. Students at this stage interact with their supervisor in varying degrees to solve problems or make decisions, and are able to make meaningful contributions as members of a health care team.

Unacceptable A substandard performance that suggests the student is making inadequate progress toward competence. An unacceptable performance is characterized by inappropriate, improper, incorrect, or unsafe actions or a lack of knowledge.

Vision of the Profession The guiding principles for the continued implementation of the profession's core values in society and for promoting, protecting, and improving the health of the public.

REFERENCES

Anderson, J. L. (1988). *The supervisory process in speech-language pathology & audiology.* Boston: Little, Brown.

Association of Canadian Occupational Therapy Regulatory Organizations (ACOTRO). (2000). *Essential competencies for occupational therapists in Canada.* Author.

Benner, P. (1982). Issues in competency-based testing. *Nursing Outlook, 30*(5), 303–309.

Bossers, A., Cook, J., Polatajko, H., & Laine, C. (1997). Understanding the role-emerging fieldwork placement. *Canadian Journal of Occupational Therapy, 64,* 70–81.

Bossers, A., Miller, L. T., Polatajko, H. J., Hartley, M., Anthony, A., & Gaiptman, B. (1998). *Competency based fieldwork evaluation for rehabilitation professionals.*

Chambers, D. W., & Glassman, P. (1997). A primer on competency-based evaluation. *Journal of Dental Education, 61*(8), 651–666.

Gage, M. (1995). Re-engineering of health care: Opportunity or threat for occupational therapists? *Canadian Journal of Occupational Therapy, 62,* 197–207.

Gaiptman, B., & Anthony, A. (1993). *Fundamentals of supervision: Leaders guide.* Toronto: Author.

Hagler, P., & McFarlane, L. (1991). Achieving maximum student potential: The supervisor as coach. *Canadian Journal of Rehabilitation, 5,* 5–16.

Landry, J. E., Hobson, S. J. G., & Polatajko, H. J. (1997). *Your guide to curriculum 2000.* School of Occupational Therapy, Faculty of Health Sciences, University of Western Ontario, 10.

London Life Insurance Company. (1994, January). *London life evaluation form.* Unpublished manuscript.

McFarlane, L., & Hagler, P. (1995, June). *Achieving maximum student potential: The supervisor as coach.* Handout presented at the clinical workshop, Toronto, ON. University of Alberta, Centre for Studies in Clinical Education.

Miller, L. T., Bossers, A., Polatajko, H. J., & Hartley, M. (2001). Development of the competency based fieldwork evaluation (CBFE). *Occupational Therapy International, 8*(4).

Neistadt, M. E. (1996). Teaching strategies for the development of clinical reasoning. *American Journal of Occupational Therapy, 50,* 676–684.

Pew Health Professions Commission. (1991, October). *Healthy America: Practitioners for the year 2005.* Author.

Prahadad, C., & Hamel, G. (1990, May–June). The core competence of the corporation. *Harvard Business Review,* 79–91.

Schön, D. (1987). *Educating the reflective practitioner.* San Francisco: Jossey-Bass.

Shippman, J. S. (2000). The practice of competency modeling. *Personal Psychology, 53*(3), 703–740.

Sullivan, T. M., & Bossers, A. (1998, May). Occupational therapy fieldwork levels. *National, The Newsletter of the Canadian Association of Occupational Therapists, 15*(3), 8–9.

COMPETENCY BASED FIELDWORK EVALUATION
For Occupational Therapists

Bossers, A., Miller, L.T., Polatajko, H.J.,
Hartley, M.

Student Evaluation

Placement History

The Competencies

1. Practice Knowledge

2. Clinical Reasoning

3. Facilitating Change with a
    Practice Process

4. Professional Interactions
    and Responsibility

5. Communication

6. Professional Development

7. Performance Management

COMPETENCY BASED FIELDWORK EVALUATION
For Occupational Therapists

Placement History

UNIVERSITY NAME: _____   Degree Granted: _____

AGENCY NAME: _____   Times Absent: _____

DATE OF PLACEMENT: _____   Times Late: _____

LENGTH OF PLACEMENT: _____   Placement Sequence: __ of __

NUMBER OF PREVIOUS FIELDWORK HOURS: _____   (i.e., placement 3 of 4)

DESCRIPTION OF PLACEMENT: _____

_____

_____

DESCRIPTION OF PROJECT (if applicable): _____

_____

MIDTERM EVALUATION

Fieldwork Educator -   Name: _____

Registration#: _____

Signature: _____

Student -   Name: _____

Signature: _____

_____ I accept this evaluation

_____ I do not accept this evaluation

FINAL EVALUATION

Fieldwork Educator -   Name: _____

Registration#: _____

Signature: _____

Student -   Name: _____

Signature: _____

_____ I accept this evaluation

_____ I do not accept this evaluation

COMPETENCY BASED FIELDWORK EVALUATION
FOR OCCUPATIONAL THERAPISTS

1. PRACTICE KNOWLEDGE

- Has the theoretical knowledge and technical expertise to serve clients/client groups, colleagues, the agency, and the profession
- Utilizes evidence based knowledge
- Knows the parameters of the profession and its role within the agency
- Understands the core values and vision of the profession

STAGES		SCORE
DEVELOPING	**1**	1 - Low Stage 1 competencies 2 - Rudimentary Stage 1 competencies 3 - Mastery of Stage 1 competencies/ Transition to Stage 2
	2	3 - Transition to Stage 2 4 - Rudimentary Stage 2 competencies 5 - Intermediate Stage 2 competencies 6 - Mastery of Stage 2 competencies/ Transition to Stage 3
	3	6 - Transition to Stage 3 7 - Rudimentary Stage 3 competencies 8 - Mastery of Stage 3 competencies/ ready to enter clinical practice

The Competency Rating Scale

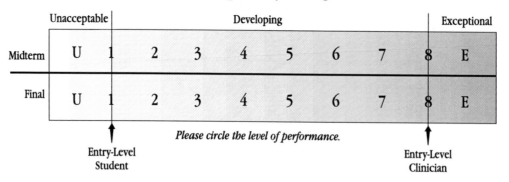

	Unacceptable				Developing					Exceptional
Midterm	U	1	2	3	4	5	6	7	8	E
Final	U	1	2	3	4	5	6	7	8	E

Please circle the level of performance.

Entry-Level Student   Entry-Level Clinician

COMMENTS:	Midterm	Final

Student's Learning Objective(s) - Practice Knowledge

Objective(s)	Resource(s) Required to Meet the Objective(s)	Evidence	Validation

The Learning Objective Rating Scale

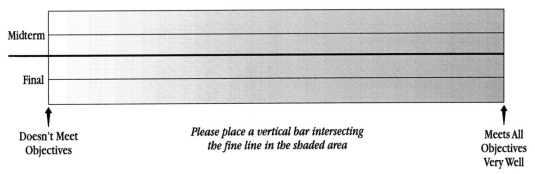

Midterm

Final

Doesn't Meet
Objectives

Please place a vertical bar intersecting the fine line in the shaded area

Meets All
Objectives
Very Well

2. CLINICAL REASONING

▸ Demonstrates analytical thinking
▸ Demonstrates conceptual thinking
▸ Demonstrates good judgment and sound decision making
▸ Utilizes good problem solving
▸ Demonstrates reasoning based on evidence

STAGES		SCORE
DEVELOPING	**1**	1 - Low Stage 1 competencies 2 - Rudimentary Stage 1 competencies 3 - Mastery of Stage 1 competencies/ Transition to Stage 2
	2	3 - Transition to Stage 2 4 - Rudimentary Stage 2 competencies 5 - Intermediate Stage 2 competencies 6 - Mastery of Stage 2 competencies/ Transition to Stage 3
	3	6 - Transition to Stage 3 7 - Rudimentary Stage 3 competencies 8 - Mastery of Stage 3 competencies/ ready to enter clinical practice

The Competency Rating Scale

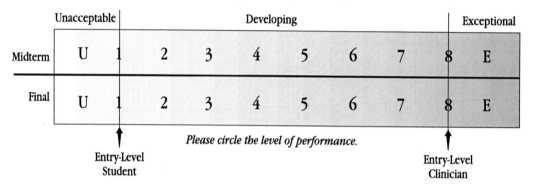

	Unacceptable	Developing	Exceptional
Midterm	U 1	2 3 4 5 6 7	8 E
Final	U 1	2 3 4 5 6 7	8 E

Please circle the level of performance.

Entry-Level Student   Entry-Level Clinician

COMMENTS: Midterm	Final

Student's Learning Objective(s) - Clinical Reasoning

Objective(s)	Resource(s) Required to Meet the Objective(s)	Evidence	Validation

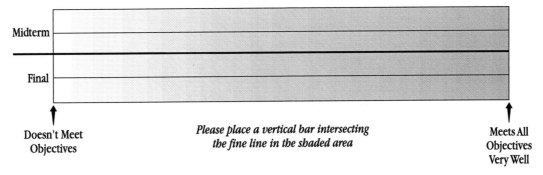

The Learning Objective Rating Scale

Midterm

Final

Doesn't Meet
Objectives

Please place a vertical bar intersecting the fine line in the shaded area

Meets All
Objectives
Very Well

3. FACILITATING CHANGE WITH A PRACTICE PROCESS

- ► Facilitates and manages change in others
- ► Establishes a therapeutic relationship
- ► Practices in a safe manner
- ► Collaboratively identifies goals
- ► Advocates and consults
- ► Practices in a client-centered manner
- ► Based on sound theory and good evidence, appropriately:
  - ► assesses needs
  - ► reports assessment results
  - ► makes referrals and plans intervention that are outcome based
  - ► carries out the intervention plan
  - ► monitors and modifies the intervention
  - ► plans and enacts the closure of the intervention
  - ► plans discharge and follow-up

STAGES		SCORE
DEVELOPING	**1**	1 - Low Stage 1 competencies 2 - Rudimentary Stage 1 competencies 3 - Mastery of Stage 1 competencies/ Transition to Stage 2
	2	3 - Transition to Stage 2 4 - Rudimentary Stage 2 competencies 5 - Intermediate Stage 2 competencies 6 - Mastery of Stage 2 competencies/ Transition to Stage 3
	3	6 - Transition to Stage 3 7 - Rudimentary Stage 3 competencies 8 - Mastery of Stage 3 competencies/ ready to enter clinical practice

The Competency Rating Scale

	Unacceptable		Developing						Exceptional
Midterm	U	1	2	3	4	5	6	7	8	E
Final	U	1	2	3	4	5	6	7	8	E

Please circle the level of performance.

Entry-Level Student

Entry-Level Clinician

COMMENTS: Midterm	Final

Student's Learning Objective(s) - Facilitating Change with a Practice Process

Objective(s)	Resource(s) Required to Meet the Objective(s)	Evidence	Validation

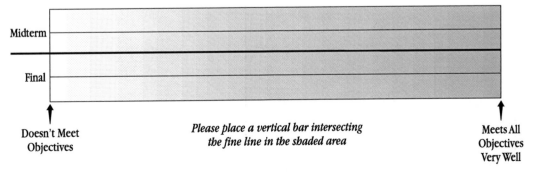

The Learning Objective Rating Scale

Midterm

Final

Doesn't Meet
Objectives

*Please place a vertical bar intersecting
the fine line in the shaded area*

Meets All
Objectives
Very Well

4. PROFESSIONAL INTERACTIONS AND RESPONSIBILITY

- ► Adheres to ethical and legal practice standards
- ► Centers on client/client group needs, always
- ► Follows through on commitments; shows respect for clients, colleagues, and the profession
- ► Contributes effectively as a team player
- ► Motivates others
- ► Fosters trust and respect as a professional
- ► Builds collaborative working relationships
- ► Deals effectively with obstacles and opposition
- ► Acts with professional integrity
- ► Gives and receives feedback effectively

STAGES		SCORE
DEVELOPING	**1**	1 - Low Stage 1 competencies 2 - Rudimentary Stage 1 competencies 3 - Mastery of Stage 1 competencies/ Transition to Stage 2
	2	3 - Transition to Stage 2 4 - Rudimentary Stage 2 competencies 5 - Intermediate Stage 2 competencies 6 - Mastery of Stage 2 competencies/ Transition to Stage 3
	3	6 - Transition to Stage 3 7 - Rudimentary Stage 3 competencies 8 - Mastery of Stage 3 competencies/ ready to enter clinical practice

The Competency Rating Scale

	Unacceptable		Developing								Exceptional
Midterm	U	1	2	3	4	5	6	7	8	E
Final	U	1	2	3	4	5	6	7	8	E

Please circle the level of performance.

Entry-Level Student ↑   ↑ Entry-Level Clinician

COMMENTS: Midterm	Final

Student's Learning Objective(s) - Professional Interactions and Responsibility

Objective(s)	Resource(s) Required to Meet the Objective(s)	Evidence	Validation

The Learning Objective Rating Scale

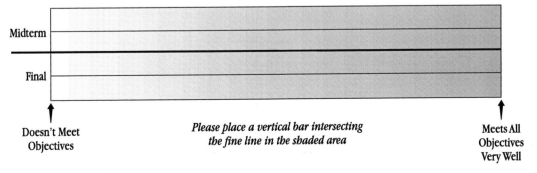

Midterm

Final

Doesn't Meet
Objectives

*Please place a vertical bar intersecting
the fine line in the shaded area*

Meets All
Objectives
Very Well

5. COMMUNICATION

- ▸ Fosters open communication
- ▸ Listens actively
- ▸ Speaks clearly and appropriately
- ▸ Listens and speaks respectfully
- ▸ Manages conflicts with diplomacy
- ▸ Provides explanations and/or education that is at an appropriate level for the client
- ▸ Writes clearly and appropriately
- ▸ Modifies language for the listener
- ▸ Uses non-verbal communication appropriately and effectively

STAGES		SCORE
DEVELOPING	**1**	1 - Low Stage 1 competencies 2 - Rudimentary Stage 1 competencies 3 - Mastery of Stage 1 competencies/ Transition to Stage 2
	2	3 - Transition to Stage 2 4 - Rudimentary Stage 2 competencies 5 - Intermediate Stage 2 competencies 6 - Mastery of Stage 2 competencies/ Transition to Stage 3
	3	6 - Transition to Stage 3 7 - Rudimentary Stage 3 competencies 8 - Mastery of Stage 3 competencies/ ready to enter clinical practice

The Competency Rating Scale

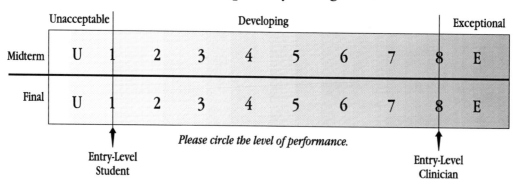

	Unacceptable				Developing					Exceptional
Midterm	U	1	2	3	4	5	6	7	8	E
Final	U	1	2	3	4	5	6	7	8	E

Please circle the level of performance.

Entry-Level
Student

Entry-Level
Clinician

COMMENTS: Midterm	Final

Student's Learning Objective(s) - Communication

Objective(s)	Resource(s) Required to Meet the Objective(s)	Evidence	Validation

The Learning Objective Rating Scale

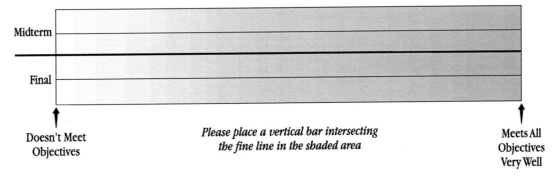

Midterm

Final

Doesn't Meet
Objectives

*Please place a vertical bar intersecting
the fine line in the shaded area*

Meets All
Objectives
Very Well

6. PROFESSIONAL DEVELOPMENT

- ▸ Demonstrates self-directed learning
- ▸ Integrates new learning into practice
- ▸ Student tries to identify areas for future growth and sets new levels for personal best
- ▸ Adapts to change
- ▸ Demonstrates commitment to the profession
- ▸ Upholds the core values of the profession
- ▸ Demonstrates skills of self-appraisal

STAGES		SCORE
DEVELOPING	**1**	1 - Low Stage 1 competencies 2 - Rudimentary Stage 1 competencies 3 - Mastery of Stage 1 competencies/ Transition to Stage 2
	2	3 - Transition to Stage 2 4 - Rudimentary Stage 2 competencies 5 - Intermediate Stage 2 competencies 6 - Mastery of Stage 2 competencies/ Transition to Stage 3
	3	6 - Transition to Stage 3 7 - Rudimentary Stage 3 competencies 8 - Mastery of Stage 3 competencies/ ready to enter clinical practice

The Competency Rating Scale

	Unacceptable		Developing							Exceptional
Midterm	U	1	2	3	4	5	6	7	8	E
Final	U	1	2	3	4	5	6	7	8	E

Entry-Level Student   *Please circle the level of performance.*   Entry-Level Clinician

COMMENTS: Midterm	Final

Student's Learning Objective(s) - Professional Development

Objective(s)	Resource(s) Required to Meet the Objective(s)	Evidence	Validation

The Learning Objective Rating Scale

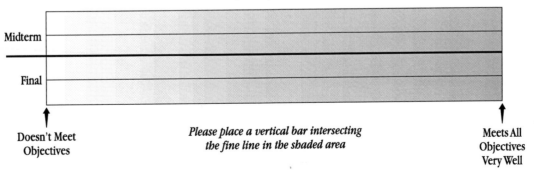

Midterm

Final

Doesn't Meet
Objectives

*Please place a vertical bar intersecting
the fine line in the shaded area*

Meets All
Objectives
Very Well

7. PERFORMANCE MANAGEMENT

- ► Self starter
- ► Completes tasks in a time efficient manner, setting priorities effectively
- ► Demonstrates effective resource utilization
- ► Demonstrates quality management
- ► Is accountable and responsible
- ► Teaches/Coaches
- ► Demonstrates operational and organizational awareness
- ► Demonstrates leadership (delegates appropriately)
- ► Seeks assistance and feedback appropriately (responds positively to constructive feedback)
- ► Demonstrates self-monitoring
- ► Organizes time and sets priorities effectively

STAGES		SCORE
DEVELOPING	**1**	1 - Low Stage 1 competencies 2 - Rudimentary Stage 1 competencies 3 - Mastery of Stage 1 competencies/ Transition to Stage 2
	2	3 - Transition to Stage 2 4 - Rudimentary Stage 2 competencies 5 - Intermediate Stage 2 competencies 6 - Mastery of Stage 2 competencies/ Transition to Stage 3
	3	6 - Transition to Stage 3 7 - Rudimentary Stage 3 competencies 8 - Mastery of Stage 3 competencies/ ready to enter clinical practice

The Competency Rating Scale

	Unacceptable		Developing							Exceptional
Midterm	U	1	2	3	4	5	6	7	8	E
Final	U	1	2	3	4	5	6	7	8	E

Please circle the level of performance.

Entry-Level Student ↑   Entry-Level Clinician ↑

COMMENTS: Midterm	Final

Student's Learning Objective(s) - Performance Management

Objective(s)	Resource(s) Required to Meet the Objective(s)	Evidence	Validation

The Learning Objective Rating Scale

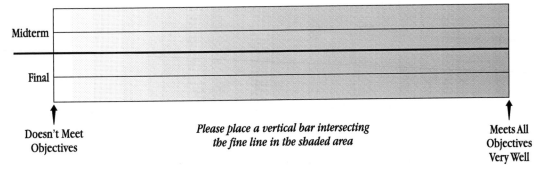

Midterm

Final

Doesn't Meet
Objectives

*Please place a vertical bar intersecting
the fine line in the shaded area*

Meets All
Objectives
Very Well

8. OVERALL RATING OF STUDENT'S PERFORMANCE

The Competency Rating Scale

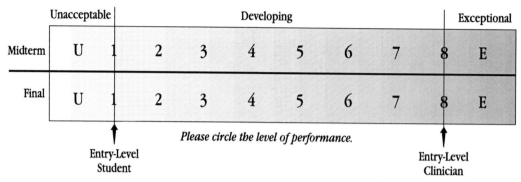

	Unacceptable				Developing					Exceptional
Midterm	U	1	2	3	4	5	6	7	8	E
Final	U	1	2	3	4	5	6	7	8	E

Please circle the level of performance.

↑ Entry-Level Student

↑ Entry-Level Clinician

COMMENTS: Midterm	Final

DIRECTIONS FOR FUTURE LEARNING:

Would you recommend the student pass this placement?   Yes ☐   No ☐

_____

Student's Name

_____

Student's Signature

_____

Date

_____

Fieldwork Educator's Name

_____

Fieldwork Educator's Signature

_____

Date

COMPETENCY BASED FIELDWORK EVALUATION
For Occupational Therapists

Bossers, A., Miller, L.T., Polatajko, H.J.,
Hartley, M.

Student Evaluation

Placement History

The Competencies

1. Practice Knowledge

2. Clinical Reasoning

3. Facilitating Change with a Practice Process

4. Professional Interactions and Responsibility

5. Communication

6. Professional Development

7. Performance Management

COMPETENCY BASED FIELDWORK EVALUATION
For Occupational Therapists

Placement History

UNIVERSITY NAME: _____

AGENCY NAME: _____

DATE OF PLACEMENT: _____

LENGTH OF PLACEMENT: _____

NUMBER OF PREVIOUS FIELDWORK HOURS: _____

DESCRIPTION OF PLACEMENT: _____
_____
_____

DESCRIPTION OF PROJECT (if applicable): _____
_____

Degree Granted: _____

Times Absent: _____

Times Late: _____

Placement Sequence: ___ of ___

(i.e., placement 3 of 4)

MIDTERM EVALUATION

Fieldwork Educator -

Name: _____

Registration#: _____

Signature: _____

Student -

Name: _____

Signature: _____

_____ I accept this evaluation

_____ I do not accept this evaluation

FINAL EVALUATION

Fieldwork Educator -

Name: _____

Registration#: _____

Signature: _____

Student -

Name: _____

Signature: _____

_____ I accept this evaluation

_____ I do not accept this evaluation

COMPETENCY BASED FIELDWORK EVALUATION
FOR OCCUPATIONAL THERAPISTS

1. PRACTICE KNOWLEDGE

- ▶ Has the theoretical knowledge and technical expertise to serve clients/client groups, colleagues, the agency, and the profession
- ▶ Utilizes evidence based knowledge
- ▶ Knows the parameters of the profession and its role within the agency
- ▶ Understands the core values and vision of the profession

STAGES		SCORE
DEVELOPING	**1**	1 - Low Stage 1 competencies 2 - Rudimentary Stage 1 competencies 3 - Mastery of Stage 1 competencies/ Transition to Stage 2
	2	3 - Transition to Stage 2 4 - Rudimentary Stage 2 competencies 5 - Intermediate Stage 2 competencies 6 - Mastery of Stage 2 competencies/ Transition to Stage 3
	3	6 - Transition to Stage 3 7 - Rudimentary Stage 3 competencies 8 - Mastery of Stage 3 competencies/ ready to enter clinical practice

The Competency Rating Scale

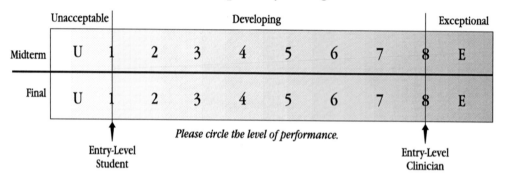

	Unacceptable			Developing						Exceptional
Midterm	U	1	2	3	4	5	6	7	8	E
Final	U	1	2	3	4	5	6	7	8	E

Please circle the level of performance.

Entry-Level Student

Entry-Level Clinician

COMMENTS: Midterm	Final

Student's Learning Objective(s) - Practice Knowledge

Objective(s)	Resource(s) Required to Meet the Objective(s)	Evidence	Validation

The Learning Objective Rating Scale

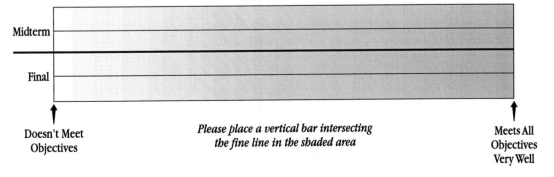

Midterm

Final

Doesn't Meet
Objectives

Please place a vertical bar intersecting the fine line in the shaded area

Meets All
Objectives
Very Well

2. CLINICAL REASONING

- ► Demonstrates analytical thinking
- ► Demonstrates conceptual thinking
- ► Demonstrates good judgment and sound decision making
- ► Utilizes good problem solving
- ► Demonstrates reasoning based on evidence

STAGES		SCORE
DEVELOPING	**1**	1 - Low Stage 1 competencies 2 - Rudimentary Stage 1 competencies 3 - Mastery of Stage 1 competencies/ Transition to Stage 2
	2	3 - Transition to Stage 2 4 - Rudimentary Stage 2 competencies 5 - Intermediate Stage 2 competencies 6 - Mastery of Stage 2 competencies/ Transition to Stage 3
	3	6 - Transition to Stage 3 7 - Rudimentary Stage 3 competencies 8 - Mastery of Stage 3 competencies/ ready to enter clinical practice

The Competency Rating Scale

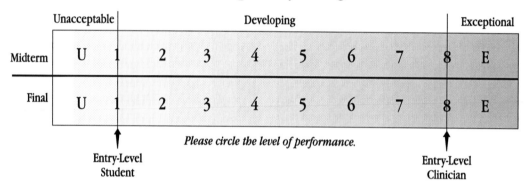

	Unacceptable				Developing					Exceptional
Midterm	U	1	2	3	4	5	6	7	8	E
Final	U	1	2	3	4	5	6	7	8	E

Please circle the level of performance.

Entry-Level Student   Entry-Level Clinician

COMMENTS: Midterm	Final

Student's Learning Objective(s) - Clinical Reasoning

Objective(s)	Resource(s) Required to Meet the Objective(s)	Evidence	Validation

The Learning Objective Rating Scale

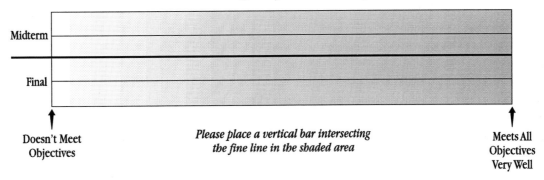

Midterm

Final

Doesn't Meet
Objectives

*Please place a vertical bar intersecting
the fine line in the shaded area*

Meets All
Objectives
Very Well

3. FACILITATING CHANGE WITH A PRACTICE PROCESS

- ▸ Facilitates and manages change in others
- ▸ Establishes a therapeutic relationship
- ▸ Practices in a safe manner
- ▸ Collaboratively identifies goals
- ▸ Advocates and consults
- ▸ Practices in a client-centered manner
- ▸ Based on sound theory and good evidence, appropriately:
  - ▸ assesses needs
  - ▸ reports assessment results
  - ▸ makes referrals and plans intervention that are outcome based
  - ▸ carries out the intervention plan
  - ▸ monitors and modifies the intervention
  - ▸ plans and enacts the closure of the intervention
  - ▸ plans discharge and follow-up

STAGES		SCORE
DEVELOPING	1	1 - Low Stage 1 competencies 2 - Rudimentary Stage 1 competencies 3 - Mastery of Stage 1 competencies/ Transition to Stage 2
	2	3 - Transition to Stage 2 4 - Rudimentary Stage 2 competencies 5 - Intermediate Stage 2 competencies 6 - Mastery of Stage 2 competencies/ Transition to Stage 3
	3	6 - Transition to Stage 3 7 - Rudimentary Stage 3 competencies 8 - Mastery of Stage 3 competencies/ ready to enter clinical practice

The Competency Rating Scale

	Unacceptable		Developing							Exceptional
Midterm	U	1	2	3	4	5	6	7	8	E
Final	U	1	2	3	4	5	6	7	8	E

Please circle the level of performance.

Entry-Level Student　　　　　　　　　　Entry-Level Clinician

COMMENTS: Midterm	Final

Student's Learning Objective(s) - Facilitating Change with a Practice Process

Objective(s)	Resource(s) Required to Meet the Objective(s)	Evidence	Validation

The Learning Objective Rating Scale

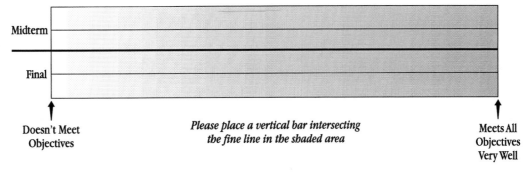

4. PROFESSIONAL INTERACTIONS AND RESPONSIBILITY

- ▸ Adheres to ethical and legal practice standards
- ▸ Centers on client/client group needs, always
- ▸ Follows through on commitments; shows respect for clients, colleagues, and the profession
- ▸ Contributes effectively as a team player
- ▸ Motivates others
- ▸ Fosters trust and respect as a professional
- ▸ Builds collaborative working relationships
- ▸ Deals effectively with obstacles and opposition
- ▸ Acts with professional integrity
- ▸ Gives and receives feedback effectively

STAGES		SCORE
DEVELOPING	**1**	1 - Low Stage 1 competencies 2 - Rudimentary Stage 1 competencies 3 - Mastery of Stage 1 competencies/ Transition to Stage 2
	2	3 - Transition to Stage 2 4 - Rudimentary Stage 2 competencies 5 - Intermediate Stage 2 competencies 6 - Mastery of Stage 2 competencies/ Transition to Stage 3
	3	6 - Transition to Stage 3 7 - Rudimentary Stage 3 competencies 8 - Mastery of Stage 3 competencies/ ready to enter clinical practice

The Competency Rating Scale

	Unacceptable		Developing							Exceptional
Midterm	U	1	2	3	4	5	6	7	8	E
Final	U	1	2	3	4	5	6	7	8	E

↑ Entry-Level Student

Please circle the level of performance.

↑ Entry-Level Clinician

COMMENTS: Midterm	Final

Student's Learning Objective(s) - Professional Interactions and Responsibility

Objective(s)	Resource(s) Required to Meet the Objective(s)	Evidence	Validation

The Learning Objective Rating Scale

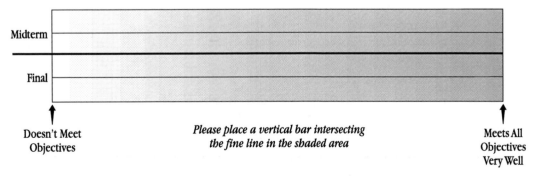

Midterm

Final

Doesn't Meet
Objectives

Please place a vertical bar intersecting the fine line in the shaded area

Meets All
Objectives
Very Well

5. COMMUNICATION

- ▸ Fosters open communication
- ▸ Listens actively
- ▸ Speaks clearly and appropriately
- ▸ Listens and speaks respectfully
- ▸ Manages conflicts with diplomacy
- ▸ Provides explanations and/or education that is at an appropriate level for the client
- ▸ Writes clearly and appropriately
- ▸ Modifies language for the listener
- ▸ Uses non-verbal communication appropriately and effectively

STAGES		SCORE
DEVELOPING	1	1 - Low Stage 1 competencies 2 - Rudimentary Stage 1 competencies 3 - Mastery of Stage 1 competencies/ Transition to Stage 2
	2	3 - Transition to Stage 2 4 - Rudimentary Stage 2 competencies 5 - Intermediate Stage 2 competencies 6 - Mastery of Stage 2 competencies/ Transition to Stage 3
	3	6 - Transition to Stage 3 7 - Rudimentary Stage 3 competencies 8 - Mastery of Stage 3 competencies/ ready to enter clinical practice

The Competency Rating Scale

	Unacceptable			Developing					Exceptional
Midterm	U	1	2	3	4	5	6	7	8	E
Final	U	1	2	3	4	5	6	7	8	E

Please circle the level of performance.

↑
Entry-Level
Student

↑
Entry-Level
Clinician

COMMENTS: Midterm	Final

Student's Learning Objective(s) - Communication

Objective(s)	Resource(s) Required to Meet the Objective(s)	Evidence	Validation

The Learning Objective Rating Scale

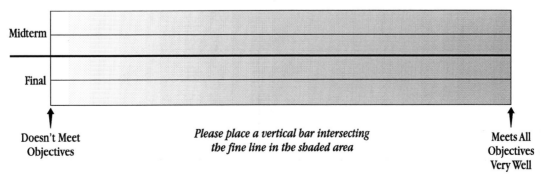

Midterm

Final

Doesn't Meet
Objectives

*Please place a vertical bar intersecting
the fine line in the shaded area*

Meets All
Objectives
Very Well

6. PROFESSIONAL DEVELOPMENT

- ► Demonstrates self-directed learning
- ► Integrates new learning into practice
- ► Student tries to identify areas for future growth and sets new levels for personal best
- ► Adapts to change
- ► Demonstrates commitment to the profession
- ► Upholds the core values of the profession
- ► Demonstrates skills of self-appraisal

STAGES		SCORE
DEVELOPING	1	1 - Low Stage 1 competencies 2 - Rudimentary Stage 1 competencies 3 - Mastery of Stage 1 competencies/ Transition to Stage 2
	2	3 - Transition to Stage 2 4 - Rudimentary Stage 2 competencies 5 - Intermediate Stage 2 competencies 6 - Mastery of Stage 2 competencies/ Transition to Stage 3
	3	6 - Transition to Stage 3 7 - Rudimentary Stage 3 competencies 8 - Mastery of Stage 3 competencies/ ready to enter clinical practice

The Competency Rating Scale

	Unacceptable	Developing							Exceptional
Midterm	U	1	2	3	4	5	6	7	8	E
Final	U	1	2	3	4	5	6	7	8	E

Please circle the level of performance.

Entry-Level Student   Entry-Level Clinician

COMMENTS: Midterm	Final

Student's Learning Objective(s) - Professional Development

Objective(s)	Resource(s) Required to Meet the Objective(s)	Evidence	Validation

The Learning Objective Rating Scale

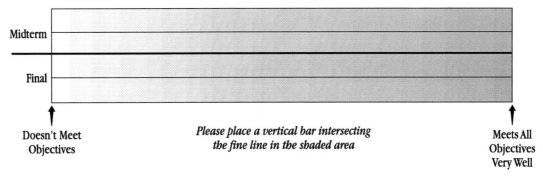

Midterm

Final

Doesn't Meet
Objectives

*Please place a vertical bar intersecting
the fine line in the shaded area*

Meets All
Objectives
Very Well

7. PERFORMANCE MANAGEMENT

- ▸ Self starter
- ▸ Completes tasks in a time efficient manner, setting priorities effectively
- ▸ Demonstrates effective resource utilization
- ▸ Demonstrates quality management
- ▸ Is accountable and responsible
- ▸ Teaches/Coaches
- ▸ Demonstrates operational and organizational awareness
- ▸ Demonstrates leadership (delegates appropriately)
- ▸ Seeks assistance and feedback appropriately (responds positively to constructive feedback)
- ▸ Demonstrates self-monitoring
- ▸ Organizes time and sets priorities effectively

STAGES		SCORE
DEVELOPING	1	1 - Low Stage 1 competencies 2 - Rudimentary Stage 1 competencies 3 - Mastery of Stage 1 competencies/ Transition to Stage 2
	2	3 - Transition to Stage 2 4 - Rudimentary Stage 2 competencies 5 - Intermediate Stage 2 competencies 6 - Mastery of Stage 2 competencies/ Transition to Stage 3
	3	6 - Transition to Stage 3 7 - Rudimentary Stage 3 competencies 8 - Mastery of Stage 3 competencies/ ready to enter clinical practice

The Competency Rating Scale

	Unacceptable		Developing							Exceptional
Midterm	U	1	2	3	4	5	6	7	8	E
Final	U	1	2	3	4	5	6	7	8	E

Please circle the level of performance.

Entry-Level Student　　　　　　　　　　　　　　　Entry-Level Clinician

COMMENTS:　　　　　　Midterm	Final

Student's Learning Objective(s) - Performance Management

Objective(s)	Resource(s) Required to Meet the Objective(s)	Evidence	Validation

The Learning Objective Rating Scale

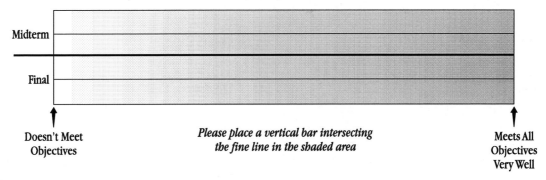

Midterm

Final

Doesn't Meet
Objectives

*Please place a vertical bar intersecting
the fine line in the shaded area*

Meets All
Objectives
Very Well

8. OVERALL RATING OF STUDENT'S PERFORMANCE

The Competency Rating Scale

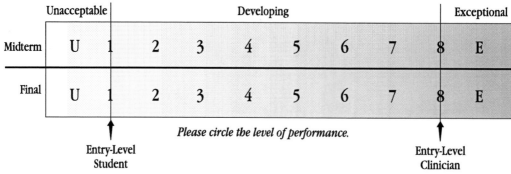

	Unacceptable		Developing							Exceptional
Midterm	U	1	2	3	4	5	6	7	8	E
Final	U	1	2	3	4	5	6	7	8	E

Please circle the level of performance.

Entry-Level Student

Entry-Level Clinician

COMMENTS: Midterm	Final

DIRECTIONS FOR FUTURE LEARNING:

Would you recommend the student pass this placement?   Yes ☐   No ☐

_____
Student's Name

_____
Student's Signature

_____
Date

_____
Fieldwork Educator's Name

_____
Fieldwork Educator's Signature

_____
Date